Nutrition, Health, Myths and All That

Frank Tennant

Published by eBookIt.com

ISBN-13: 978-1-4566-2447-7

Contents

PREFACE

"Every sentence that I utter should be regarded by you not as an assertion but as a question."

This is how Niels Bohr, the Nobel prize winning physicist, often started his lectures. I don't pretend to be in his league but, in similar vein, my objective is to fill your head with questions so that on taking responsibility for your health, you make your own best decisions.

To stimulate those questions I will summarise the knowledge I have acquired on nutrition, as it relates to health, in the last fifty years and in particular the last thirty. Parts of this information are my own views, which may be contrary to conventional thinking, and some is supported by research, which can become outdated.

Stephen Hawking in 'A Brief History of Time' wrote: *In effect, we have redefined the task of science to be the discovery of laws that will enable us to predict events up to the limits set by the uncertainty principle.*

My observation is that much of the so-called knowledge on Nutrition that has been bandied around in the last few decades has led us off track. There have been many red herrings and it is an area where there is so much to learn yet it appears the uncertainty principle has been ignored by many determined to claim certainty. It is also an area in which the German physicist, Max Planck's statement is very relevant: *A new scientific truth does not triumph by convincing its opponents and making them see the light, but rather because its opponents eventually die, and a new generation grows up that is familiar with it.*

Some conventional thinking on nutrition might take a generation or more to be superseded.

It is more than fifty years since I was first made aware of the link between our health and the health of the soil from which we obtain our food.

In retrospect, I was fortunate, when studying Agricultural Science, to get to know one of the early pioneers of organic farming in England. He was in his 70's at the time and had already written two books on the subject and was completing his third one. His books are still being used by organic farmers around the world. He sparked my questioning of modern agricultural methods, though it took me years of reading, observation and experience to really understand the implications. He and his fellow colleagues were originally know as 'muck and magic' or 'humus' farmers. These days they may be grouped as practicing organic, sustainable, biological or ecological farming. There are differences between them but in essence they rely on what I was originally advised "A healthy soil produces healthy plants which influence the health of the people and animals that eat them". As far as our health is concerned humus farmers, as you will learn, is the most appropriate description.

I was advised to read a book called "The Stuff Man's Made Of" . Let me quote you the summary on the inside of the dust cover and at the end you will understand why I suggest you read on:

"Never before have the people of the West enjoyed such abundant food, so much medical care, such freedom from epidemics. Yet they are increasingly susceptible to cancer, arteriosclerosis, heart disease, arthritis, gastric ulcers and many other functional disorders. These diseases are degenerative, coming from within and striking all ages. What is happening?

......a handful of research scientists, working apart, nevertheless reached certain common conclusions - that health is a positive process profoundly influenced by food and environment; that there is a nutritional cycle comprising soil, plants, animals and human beings, impairment of which at any point may impair health at other points; that the basis of positive health is wholesome food raised from biologically fertile soil.

This concept, though still too revolutionary for official acceptance, has been strengthened by subsequent work and experience. It is interesting a growing number of intelligent people in all walks of life. It may represent a great contribution to the conquest of degenerative disease".

This summary reads like today's situation yet that book was published in 1959.

It is a summary of information from the first half of the last century which shows the link between modern agricultural practices, food manufacturing and the incidence of degenerative diseases. I first read it in the early 1960's.

The author noted some interesting statistics.

In the first half of the last century improved public health reduced the deaths from infectious diseases by 90%, at the same time deaths from degenerative diseases increased by 90%.

So, this is not new knowledge. It has been known for some time but the problems have escalated.

Let me, however, start at the beginning.

EVOLUTION AND FOOD

It can take many thousand years of evolution for our biochemistry to manage some foods we are currently encouraged to eat. Hopefully we may wake up to this fact and stop eating them or, possibly, by a process of selection many may cease being able to breed and those that are left could be the progenitors of a new species of homo sapiens!

To give us an indication of beneficial foods it is important to understand what we ate as we evolved.

Opinions differ as to when the present version of homo sapiens, our ancestors, emerged. It seems to have been somewhere between 125,000 and 700,000 years ago.

Our closest living 'relative', the chimpanzee, diverted from our mutual family tree some 5 million years ago. But there are only 1.6% of genes that separate us from them - a very small genetic distance. The main changes have been morphological - to the surface! Our biochemistry remains the same. Maybe they can give us some clues as to what is a healthy diet.

There are those who propose that we should not eat meat as our ancestors were basically vegetarian. Yet, some 5 million years ago we had a cousin (*australopithelus robustus*), descended from *ramapithecus*, our common ancestor. *Robustus* was vegetarian but that line died out.

There is much evidence to show that our forbearers (*australopithelus africanus*) ate plenty of fish and fowls and that, 2 million years ago, they used stone tools to cut up meat.

Meat has a more concentrated supply of protein than plants. Eating meat, therefore, cuts down the bulk and the time spent in eating by two thirds. The author of 'The Ascent of Man' Dr Jan Bronowski, rates this extra time as the spur that enabled our forbearers to move from the biological evolution of man to the next 2 million years of cultural evolution - the making of tools and various art forms which led us, 12,000 years ago, into the Agricultural Revolution.

Our Stone Age ancestors ate three times the amount of protein that we do; half the fat; six times the fibre; two to three times the calcium; and no sugar - apart from the occasional honey.

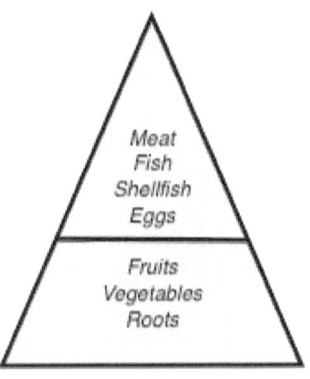

The Stone Age Food Pyramid as designed by Dr Philip Goscienski

Meat
Fish
Shellfish
Eggs

Fruits
Vegetables
Roots

Over many millennia, mankind learnt through trial, error and instinct which foods were beneficial. Animals still have this instinct yet homo sapiens seems to have lost it. As I walk across the paddocks with my dog I notice that at certain times of the year she will eat certain grasses. Livestock will often eat what we may term weeds - they seem to know that they need what that particular plant has to offer.

There is evidence that 14,000 years ago, people living on the islands we now refer to as Japan, were experimenting with cooking food and learning which combinations worked best. They used fire and clay pots.

In recent years the microwave has been a boon to our fast lifestyles...or has it? Has it been in use long enough for us to know? More on that later.

It seems that our nutritional problems started with the Agricultural Age.

NUTRITION AND DISEASE

The WHO (World Health Organisation) has not been able to find a degenerative disease that is not linked to nutrition.

The 'Agricultural Age' commenced in the Fertile Crescent of present-day Iraq about 12,000 years ago. In South America it started 5000 years ago and in Northern Europe some 2000 years after that. We have not had time to adapt to these rapid changes.

In 1788 the agricultural age started in Australia. We can see the deleterious effects of this to the health of the aboriginal peoples. This has compounded in the last hundred years with the advent of food processing.

Dr.Philip Goscienski, author of "Health Secrets of the Stone Age", writes: *Since the beginning of the Agricultural Revolution ...... not even an eye-blink within the cosmos .... our body chemistry has not had time to adapt to foods such as processed cereal grains and dairy products. It's even less likely for us to have adapted to the foods that have become available in the past few generations.*

When cereal grains replaced fruits, vegetables and animal protein, the average persons stature diminished by several centimetres and his lifespan by several years. Infant mortality climbed. Bone and tooth disorders increased as did infectious diseases and iron deficiency anaemia. In addition we lost 10% of our brains.

Oral health influences our overall health. DNA samples show that 5000 years before the Agricultural Revolution reached Northern Europe the bacterial ecosystem found in the mouths of our meat-eating ancestors benefited from diversity. Since the start of the Agricultural Revolution there has been a decrease of between 30-40% in this rate of diversity with a much greater representation of disease-causing bacteria. Apart from the mouth oral bacteria is also associated with diabetes, heart disease and some cancers.

Heart disease was first diagnosed in 1908. Now one in three Australians suffer from heart disease, diabetes, and, or cancer. This is apart from problems like alzheimer's, dementia, autism, chronic fatigue syndrome amongst other degenerative ills.

What's happened?

Let me remind you of the summary from "The Stuff Mans' Made Of": *'the incidence of degenerative diseases can be linked to modern agricultural practices and food manufacturing'.*

As a result of these practices it has been estimated that some foods currently contain as little as 20% of the nutrition available to our ancestors three or four generations ago.

For many decades numerous diets have been introduced to attempt a remedy for this increase in degenerative diseases. One of these was the low fat diet.

This diet was originated by a Dr Ancel Keys. As a result of his population studies he claimed there was a link between heart disease and saturated fat consumption. We have also been advised that reducing saturated fat consumption is necessary to reduce weight.

However, when I looked at the Australian statistics I found that since the start of the low fat diet the incidence of cardiovascular diseases had nearly trebled, deaths from cancer had increased by a third and we are experiencing an obesity epidemic.

It did not seem credible that there could be a link between saturated fats and heart disease.

Even though Ancel Key's research has been shown to be badly flawed the low fat diet continues to be promoted.

During an ABC interview in August 2011 a professor with expertise in nutrition quoted a recent fifteen year study which showed there was no link between saturated fats and heart disease. Yet in the same breath he advised against using coconut oil - presumably because of its 'saturated fat content'. More on that later.

I then looked at food consumption in Australia to find out what may have changed: In the last half of the last century, sugar in manufactured foods doubled; the consumption of vegetable oils increased by 84% and butter consumption slumped to a fifth of what it had been 70 years before; the consumption of fizzy drinks almost trebled and breakfast foods increased by 60% with a surge in the last 20 years.

Breakfast foods have a high level of sugar and the level in fizzy drinks is, what one might call, toxic.

During this period the consumption of beef, a major source of saturated fats, dropped 40%.

This indicated to me that our health problems were more likely to be linked to sugar and vegetable oils than saturated fats.

Let's examine how this has influenced food manufacturers.

FOOD MANUFACTURING

Vegetable Oils

Margarine, made from vegetable oils, was invented at the end of the 19th century and marketed in the early part of last century as a poor man's butter.

Food manufacturers and the vegetable oil industry took advantage of the low fat diet to promote the use of vegetable oils as a replacement for butter, lard, some tropical oils and other saturated fats. These vegetable fats and oils were used to produce salad dressings, biscuits, pastries, snack foods and fried foods.

The hydrogenation process made it possible to create cheap fats and oils that were resistant to heat and rancidity. These were low cost good tasting substitutes for the traditional fats. But the nutritional qualities of these new fats and oils are different from the ones they replaced:

- Omega-3 has been reduced
- Omega-6 has risen to record levels
- A group, known as trans fatty acids (TFA's), or synthetic fats, have been introduced to the human diet for the first time in large quantities. They damage cell membranes and are linked to heart disease and cancer.

Both the lopsided ratio of omega-6 to omega-3 and the man-made synthetic fats have had a profoundly negative effect on human health.

Insufficient or disproportionate amounts of Essential Fatty Acid (EFA's— Omega-3 & Omega-6) in our diet can have a devastating effect on the nervous system. This influences the development of the brain in foetuses, infants, and children. It can cause mood problems such as violence, aggression, social isolation and self-mutilation. (*Appendix B for more information*)

A Healthy ratio of omega-3 to omega-6 is between 1:1 and 1:3. Many vegetable oils have an excess of omega-6 Essential Fatty Acids: soy is 1:7, corn 1:57 and sunflower 1:71. Olive oil, on the other hand is 1:3.

The hunter gatherer consumed a ratio of 1:1.

It is estimated that we now, on average, consume 1 part omega-3 to over 20 parts omega-6.

The reduction in the size of our brains since the start of the Agricultural Age is likely linked to insufficient consumption of omega-3. It has been identified as the most serious nutritional deficiency in the Western Diet.

Let's take a look at another culprit.

Sugar

The fructose component of sugar, which makes up about half any sugar declared on labels, has been linked to obesity, type 2 diabetes, heart disease and cancer.

You might ask "what about the fructose in fruit?" The fibre in the fruit helps to counteract the problem but our early ancestors would not have eaten a lot of fruit and certainly would not have drunk fruit juice whence the fibre has been removed.

Our genes remember a 'sugar hit'.

Australian research has found that genes remember a sugar hit for two weeks. Prolonged poor eating habits are capable of permanently altering DNA. A study on human heart tissue and mice showed that a sugar hit switches off genetic controls designed to protect the body against diabetes and heart disease. The chocolate bar you ate this morning can have very acute effects, and those effects can continue up to two weeks. These changes continue beyond the meal itself and have the ability to alter natural metabolic responses to diet. Regular poor eating habits amplify the effect, with genetic damage lasting months or years and potentially passing through bloodlines.

It's in our early years that we develop our eating habits and tastes. A friend's grand-daughter had very little sugar in the first four years of her life. Now, at the age of nine she prefers a savoury or a piece of fruit in preference to cake. When visiting friends she often comments that the food was 'too sweet'.

Research in Sweden indicates that once a youth is obese the fat cells are conditioned and the situation is very likely irreversible.

However, being at an optimal weight, does not necessarily mean one is healthy.

Seneca, the 'wise Greek', is reputed to have been the first man to use the phrase 'everything in moderation'. As far as refined sugar is concerned we have ignored his wisdom. He would have eaten whole foods.

Whole Foods

We evolved eating whole foods and combinations of whole foods.

As in so much of nature many of these have a synergistic effect - the many nutrients in a food compliment each other so making the whole much more beneficial. Amongst other things food manufacturing has destroyed this synergy.

Let's take flour as an example.

By converting wholemeal flour into white flour we lose 80% of the nutrition. We are left with an anti-nutrient. It takes more energy for us to digest the white bread than the energy it supplies. Don't be fooled by the fact that some labels tell you they have added back a few of the nutrients - why did they remove them in the first place and why don't they put them all back?

> *The whiter your bread*
> *The sooner you're dead*
>
> Old Scottish Saying

Another example is milk.

Cow's milk is one of the most nourishing of foods when it is raw.

There are some parts of the world where the inhabitants are known for their longevity and a major part of their diets are raw cow's milk and products produced from that milk. But pasteurised milk does not appear to have the same nutritional value as raw milk.

Why is milk pasteurised?

It was introduced to prevent the spread of diseases in particular TB. But with modern methods of hygiene and TB testing this problem has been solved. Raw milk is better for your health than pasteurised. It is certainly more nourishing.

Researchers analysing the diet and health of 4700 primary school children in England, found that those who lived on farms had significantly fewer symptoms of asthma, hay fever and eczema. They looked at many factors that could have had an influence on this and found that the greatest benefits came from drinking raw milk. They concluded that even relatively infrequent exposure to unpasteurised milk was sufficient to have a protective effect. Just a couple of glasses a week reduced a child's chances of developing eczema by almost 40% and hay fever by 10%.

Dr. Evelyn Sprawson, of London Hospital, stated that children in the institution in which he worked who were fed on raw milk had perfect teeth, whereas others in circumstances identical in all respects except that their milk was pasteurised, had defective teeth. *The Medical Testament 1939.*

Pasteurised milk has been linked to a wide range of health problems. *(Appendix A).*

However, over some thousands of years our ancestors worked out how to make grains and milk more digestible.

Fermentation

The only milk available in the Stone Age came from lactating human females, and none was available after the first 2 to 4 years of life. It is only recently that 'foreign' foods like cows milk and grains have become part of our diets.

A significant number of people do not tolerate dairy products. In most people the digestive enzyme, lactase, declines with age and, in some population groups it is absent in about 80% of them after the age of six. However, our forbearers worked out that if these foods were fermented they would be more digestible.

Grains contain phytic acid which inhibit enzymes that we need for digestion and also reduce the absorption of certain minerals and affect vitamin D metabolism. This problem can be reduced by soaking the grains or eating sourdough bread which contains lactic acid that breaks down the phytates.

Raw milk is more digestible than the pasteurised variety because it contains more enzymes that help to break it down. Many people who are lactose intolerant can drink sour milk or eat yoghurt because these fermented products have been pre-digested by microbes and the lactase has been converted to lactic acid.

Let's examine another example of what happens when food is "manufactured" or "processed".

Processed Foods

Sir Robert McCarrison, C.I.E., M.D., F.R.C.P. carried out an experiment on young rats. One group were fed on a diet similar to that of the healthy peoples of Northern India and the other on a diet in common use by many people in England.

The rats on the Northern Indian diet grew well, there was little disease amongst them and they lived happily together.

Those fed on the 'English diet' did not grow well, many became ill and the stronger ones began to kill and eat the weaker. They suffered from diseases of the lungs, stomach and intestines, and nerves. These were diseases from which one in every three people in England suffered.

Dr Francis Pottenger published research in a book called "Pottenger's Cats". He monitored the progress of 900 cats over three generations to help determine the effect of diet upon their health. One group of animals was fed raw meat and milk while a second group received just processed food, including pasteurised milk and processed meat and fish. The group fed with nothing but processed food declined at an alarming rate and the problems were magnified in each generation, to the point that the third generation was horrifically handicapped. Many of the kittens were born dead and those that survived could barely walk and died within weeks.

Could this be an indication of where we are heading?

What about the effect of modern agricultural practices on our nutrition and health?

MODERN AGRICULTURAL PRACTICES

Most modern agricultural practices have been based on controlling rather than working with nature.

The aim of modern agriculture has been to increase the production per hectare which has been achieved to the detriment of the nutritional value per hectare. Plant breeding has focussed on producing good looking produce that is early ripening and has a high yield. No consideration has been given to their nutritional value.

'Artificial' fertilisers, insecticides, fungicides and herbicides have been used to increase yields per hectare without taking into account or realising, at the time, the longer term damage this does to the land and the ecology as well as the shorter term damage done to the nutritional value of the crops.

We should also heed the residual effects of the chemicals used in agriculture.

A WHO study of 700 rural and 700 urban families found that they all had unacceptable levels of 18 farm chemicals.

There are many pesticides commonly used in Australia that have been banned in the EU.

Healthy Plants

A healthy plant will transfer its attributes to the animals and humans that consume it. At the same time its healthy immune system is better able to withstand diseases and insects. Professor Phil Callahan has discovered that plants put out a signal in the infra red part of the spectrum. If a plant is sick or deficient in nutrients, it puts out a signal which attracts insects. This is part of the cycle where insects are the garbage collectors. By killing the insects we protect and eat the sick plants!

But, for a plant to be healthy it needs a healthy soil.

A study underwritten by a major bank came to the conclusion that the amount of organic matter in the soil is the single most important factor to influence success in farming. This humus also retains large amounts of water so contributing to drought resistance. Yet for many years modern agricultural methods have ignored the importance of maintaining a high level of humus - short term it has not been deemed important.

A healthy soil is biologically active. It has a fine mineral and microbial balance. The soil is a living entity composed of insects, worms, protozoa, bacteria and fungi with threads of mycelia linking plant roots and working their way down to deepen the top soil. These feed off the humus and each other. A healthy soil breathes - oxygen moves in and carbon dioxide moves to the plants which use it in photosynthesis.

In regard to mycelia, Friend Sykes, one of the founders of the UK Soil Association in the 1940's, states in his third book - Modern Humus Farming - *"80% of agricultural crops are known to be mycorrhiza-formers........... The white threads of mycelium contribute enormously to the growth of the plant, for apart from the fact that they are a living bridge through which the plant can draw its nutriment, they are themselves a living substance, food for the soil, as well as for the host plant itself...*

Any soil which is not forming mycorrhiza is in bad condition. This can only be remedied by the application of humus, artificial fertilisers being lethal to mycorrhizal formation."

The worm is probably the most important contributor to a biologically healthy soil.

In 1837 Charles Darwin presented a paper on moulds in which he concluded that all vegetable moulds pass many times through the intestinal canals of worms.

A study has shown that inorganic fertilisers (such as nitrogen and phosphate) kill worms. Modern agricultural practices have contributed to the destruction of soil fertility.

Friend Sykes gives an account of visiting two neighbouring gardens. One had been farmed using properly decomposed compost whereas the second had used some un-decomposed horse manure and artificial fertilisers.

In the first section were "*hundreds of fine threads of mycelium......the soil underneath was a mass of them and you could trace them to the surface and back again into the stem of the plant...........an example of what is known as mycorrhizal association - in other words the 'living bridge' which Nature provides for the conducting of the sap and solutions of nutriment in the soil through a tubular or cellular thread to the plant......these threads of mycelium..... function as a great feeder of the crop*".

In the second section "*there were no threads of mycelium anywhere to be seen, and the quality of the fruit as well as the weight of it, was not to be compared with that in the first section, although the botanical variety in both cases was the same*".

What is evident is that you cannot have healthy plants without mycorrhizae and these only exist in biologically fertile soils. It has been estimated that the symbiotic relationship between plants and mycorrhizae can increase the effective root area by ten to a thousand times. Colin Tudge in "The Secret Life of Trees" points out that these mycorrhizae can cover several hectares.

The knowledge of mycelia is not recent. In fact Professor Frank of Berlin, whilst studying truffles in the 1880's, first identified and named these structures. Yet, proponents of 'scientific agricultural practices' have ignored them.

There is now an increasing understanding of the importance of worms and mycelia as contributors to a biologically fertile soil.

> "Food is the agent of transfer of the soil's qualities into the bodies of man and beast."
> E.B.Balfour

Keeping in mind the importance of the structure and biological activity required in a healthy soil it amazes me that there is a belief one can produce healthy nutritious plants by growing them hydroponically.

The BRIX scale is a method used to measure the nutritional density of plants. Nutritionally rich food should read 12+ which is the level at which plants have begun to resist insects and diseases. Hydroponics seem to range between 1½ and 3 although I have seen a claim of 6 on a vegetable grown by one hydroponic farm.

I checked the Brix scale of a very red, truss, hydroponically grown tomato. It came out at 4 which is considered poor. On the other hand a normal commercially grown Roma tomato which was still a bit green and yellow at one end came out at 6 which is considered average for a tomato.

On another occasion I compared the commercially (normal) grown vegetables with those labelled as 'organic' from the same supermarket. Here is the result (I have also indicated what a good and excellent level is for those vegetables):

	Normal	Organic	Good	Excellent
Tomato	7	5	8	12
Carrot	6	9	12	18
Broccoli	5	5	10	12
Pink Lady Apple	13	16	14	18
Lemon	8	10*	8	12
* This came from my lemon tree which has only had some blood and bone added over the years				

As you can see from the above, 'organic' does not necessarily indicate that it is nutritionally superior. In this sample of the tomatoes it is less so. The reason is that organic may be chemical free but it does not necessarily mean it has been grown in a biologically fertile soil.

I left the carrots in the above sample on my kitchen bench for five days. By then the ones with the Brix 6 reading were covered in mould. Those with the Brix 9 reading were mould free.

What about livestock?

Livestock

Ruminants evolved eating grasses. Yet we have been feeding grain to fatten them and improve milk production. What does that do to the end product that we consume?

There is a major difference in the nutritional value of butter, milk and beef from grass-fed as opposed to grain-fed cattle (*Appendix A*).

There is also a difference in the nutritional value of the grasses or the hay made from them.

It has been shown that cattle grazing in biologically fertile paddocks can consume half as much bulk, yet, produce more milk with higher butterfat and are healthier than those grazing paddocks which have been treated according to modern agricultural practices.

What about the livestock that are fed antibiotics to improve their feed to weight conversion rates?

What do these antibiotics do to the flora in their stomachs and so their general health *(more on this in the section on the germ theory)*? How much of these do we have to eat over a period for our health to be affected? Have the regulators got the right formula?

Then there is a possible adverse outcome in breeding dairy cattle for high milk yields.

Two types of milk have been identified and designated as A1 and A2. The difference is in one of 209 amino acids which results in A1 milk being linked to a range of diseases and mental disorders. The A1 milk tends to be produced by high yielding dairy cattle so there has been a trend to move towards these. *(Appendix A)*.

How do genetically modified (GM) crops affect our health?

Genetically Modified Crops
Could the sort of GM crops being produced these days occur naturally?

Plants do cross-fertilise. Wheat is a good example.

After the last ice-age wild wheat crossed with goat grass to produce emmer which had a much plumper head. This was probably the first variety that was cultivated by our ancestors.

Emmer then crossed with another goat grass with a still larger head which is bread wheat. But this ear is too tight and will never spread in the wind like earlier varieties. This bread wheat can only multiply with help - man must harvest the ear and scatter the seeds. This mutation came about at the start of the Agricultural Revolution.

Since then mankind has produced more and more productive hybrids of wheat by crossing various strains. Our modern plant contains over twice the number of genes of the earlier varieties. We may not have evolved fast enough to cope with these extra genes. Maybe this accounts for some of the allergies associated with wheat.

But crossing different strains of wheat is hardly the same as introducing a 'foreign' gene to make the plant resistant to an herbicide.

There is more and more evidence of allergic reactions to such GM crops.

Pharmaceutical companies who plan to introduce a medicament for human use have to justify their claims and its safety by producing copious research findings some of which are on humans. Yet, a GM crop for human consumption does not require any such proof. Is that because it is classed as a food and not a medicine? Yet both are consumed by humans.

An editorial in a world leading medical journal, the Lancet, said "it is astounding that the U.S Food and Drug Administration has not changed their stance on genetically modified food adopted in 1992 which states that they do not believe it is 'necessary to conduct comprehensive scientific reviews of foods derived from bioengineered plants.' The editorial continued "this stance is taken despite good reasons to believe that specific risks may exist....Governments should never have allowed these products into the food chain without insisting on rigorous testing for effects on health. The companies should have paid greater attention to the possible risks to health......"

The GM situation might best be summarised by Thierry Vrain, a former research scientist for Agriculture Canada, who at one stage was most enthusiastic about the benefits of GM crops:

"Not only are GM foods less nutritious than non-GM foods, they pose distinct health risks, are inadequately regulated, harm the environment and farmers, and are a poor solution to world hunger. Worse still, these questionable GM crops are now polluting non-GM crops, leading to contamination that cannot ever be "recalled" the way you can take a bad drug off the market ... once traditional foods are contaminated with GM genes, there is no going back!" (Appendix F).

This leads me to another subject. How much credence should we give to pronouncements by experts?

EXPERTS

The human race has made remarkable advances through scientific research. I do not propose to denigrate that. I wish, however, to make you aware that expert opinions should not be treated as sacrosanct irrespective of whom the expert is. If it does not make sense in the bigger picture, in what we understand of nature, then look for another answer.

Winston Churchill once described the qualifications desirable in a prospective politician. I think it is also an apt description of many experts: "The ability to foretell what is going to happen tomorrow, next week, next month, and next year. And to have the ability afterwards to explain why it didn't happen."

Richard Feynman, the Nobel prize-winning physicist, wrote: "There is an expanding frontier of ignorance." In other words the more we learn the more we realise how much there is to learn.

But many "experts" do not appreciate their limitations - they restrict themselves by their own expertise.

In 'The Living Soil' E.B. Balfour discusses the fragmentation of research. "Whatever we study, our tendency is to break it up into little bits, thereby destroying the whole, and then to study the effect of our behaviour of the separate pieces as though they were independent , instead of - as in fact they are - interdependent."

The following account gives a graphic example of this:

A French arborist was studying trees in the Amazon rain forest. One day his Indian assistant, pointing to a frog, asked him "Do you know about this frog?"

The arborist replied: "No, I am an expert in trees."

The Indian then explained how the life cycle of the tree and frog were interdependent......the trees were only part of the lifecycle of the forest as a whole.

When, like the Frenchman, we lose touch with the bigger picture then we lose some understanding.......... understanding which may adversely affect our decisions.

Let me give some examples of symbiosis to illustrate that one cannot take one plant or animal (or even human) in isolation to understand the whole.

The canopy of a large tree contains more creatures than the whole population of New York. These creatures are interdependent and the tree is part of a forest that has a symbiotic relationship with other trees, plants and fungi. A single fungal mycelium, sometimes covering several hectares may connect with many different trees in a form of cooperative feeding.

Broad beans communicate with each other. If one is attacked by aphids it sends a message to the others through fungal hyphae in the soil. This alerts them to release a volatile chemical that repels aphids and attracts aphid-hunting wasps.

Similarly tomatoes have a symbiotic relationship with the hyphae of soil fungi who provide them with minerals in exchange for food. When one plant is infected by leaf blight nearby plants start activating genes that help ward off the infection. The message about the leaf blight may also be transmitted through the hyphae.

Nature is replete with synergisms and symbiosis. Later I shall point out how synergisms within the plants themselves affect our nutrition.

Experts can be so focussed on their area of expertise they lose sight of the whole picture. This is particularly so where nature is involved.

Sometimes conventional thought is so powerful anything to the contrary is unacceptable.

30% of all scientific papers that have been peer reviewed and published in reputable scientific journals are subsequently proved to be incorrect. Much of this is shown to be caused by what I might politely refer to as 'human weaknesses'.

Richard Horton, editor of *Lancet, once stated: "We know the system of peer review is biased, unjust, unaccountable, incomplete, easily fixed, often insulting, usually ignorant, occasionally foolish, and frequently wrong."*

In September 2000 UK's *Times Higher Education Supplement* published the results of a poll of 500 scientists 30% of whom claimed that their financial sponsor had asked them to change their research conclusions. "The figure included 17% who had been asked to change their conclusions to suit their sponsor's preferred outcome, 10% who said they had been asked to do so to obtain further contracts and 3% who claimed they had been asked to make changes to discourage publication." This, of course, only included those scientists who were prepared to admit they had succumbed to pressure.

Recently *The Economist* in a briefing on research reported that scientists at Amgen, a drug company, tried to replicate 53 studies that they considered landmarks in the basic science of cancer. They were only able to reproduce the original results in six of the fifty-three.

Consider the case of aspartame, the artificial sweetener:

Of the 165 peer-reviewed studies conducted on it by 1995 the results were evenly divided between those that found no problem and those that raised questions about the sweetener's safety. Of the studies that found no problem all were paid for by the manufacturer of the sweetener. All the studies financed by non-industry and non-government sources raised questions. Aspartame is the main sweetener used in diet drinks and is designated by code number 951.

When research linked trans fats to heart disease the US Department of Agriculture arranged for all margarines to be tested for trans fats. Every brand contained disturbingly high levels. The scientist in charge of the testing attempted to publish his findings in a scientific journal but the USDA refused to allow the information to be published. The USDA was protecting the food industry - not the health of the nation.

There are times when the advice of experts influences health departments and governments to promote a solution which causes problems over and above the one they were attempting to solve.

Let me give you some examples:

Low Fat Diet

I have mentioned the damage caused by the low fat diet. Even though many years ago Ancel Keys's studies were shown to be flawed we are still left with the original thinking which is heavily promoted throughout the world. The vegetable oil industry had taken advantage of this and further conditioned people's minds to the evils of saturated fats. The result is the scourge of trans fatty acids (TFAs) and the problems they have caused to our health. It has also deprived us of many of the benefits of, for instance, full cream milk.

Pasteurisation and homogenisation of milk are another sad saga in this respect.

Another 'hang-over' from this is the advice to avoid coconut oil because it contains a form of saturated fat. Yet this product has been consumed by generations of peoples in many parts of the world without any deleterious effects. It is known to build up the immune system. It is from the perennial nuts, those grown on trees, that mankind has over the years selected what is beneficial. The more recent annual crops of nuts, such as canola (rape), sunflower, safflower and peanuts, from which many vegetable oils are pressed are really unknown in regard to their longterm effects. We do know that most of these vegetable oils that we buy from the supermarket are at least partially hydrogenated and many have high levels of Omega-6. These, as I have mentioned, are causing health problems.

Sun Exposure

When there was evidence that excessive exposure to the sun caused melanoma we were encouraged to slip, slop, slap and protect ourselves from the sun's rays. But our forbearers were exposed to the sun all and every day of their lives. We have evolved exposed to the sun so it would surely be beneficial even though excessive exposure by fair skinned people in Australia may cause problems.

A major source of our Vitamin D comes from the sun's UV rays acting with a precursor chemical located in our skin. It is unlikely that this is the same D that is ingested from plants or supplements. I cannot see the evolution of two such different sources producing the same Vitamin D. The lack of this vitamin, if 'vitamin' is a correct description, is being linked to more and more diseases - poor immune systems, multiple sclerosis, depression, type 1 diabetes, cardiovascular disease, dementia, fractures, rheumatoid arthritis, inflammation, schizophrenia, parkinson, stroke, epilepsy and sixteen types of cancer including melanoma, the main skin cancer that initially spurred the slip, slap, slop campaign! There is also evidence that exposure to sunlight lowers blood pressure and benefits your cardiovascular system. This benefit alone may outweigh the potential skin cancer risk. *(See appendix H for a solution).*

There is now evidence that sunshine's benefits go well beyond Vitamin D. It has pain-killing properties, increases subcutaneous fat metabolism, regulates our lifespan (solar cycles appear to be able to directly affect the human genome, thereby influencing lifespan), improves evening alertness, and it seems we may absorb energy directly from the sun, like plants do. In addition UVB exposure has been shown to enhance mood and energy, affect melatonin regulation, suppress MS symptoms, and treat skin diseases

Like the low fat diet, here is another case of experts focussing on one small area - preventing sunburn. Governments and their health departments are then persuaded to promote their findings without thinking about the effect this might have on the bigger picture.

Regulatory authorities are designed to protect our health and in the main are effective in doing so. However, one does wonder if they are sometimes over influenced by groups that may have another agenda. Let me give you some examples:

Regulatory Authorities

It is estimated that an average Australian consumes five kilograms of food additives each year. The good news is that most of these are considered to be quite safe….however…some 50 of these 'approved' chemical additives are known to cause behavioural changes in children & adolescents. Many of these additives are known to cause severe allergic reactions including rashes, headaches, migraines & asthma. Some of these are prohibited in other countries as being suspected or known carcinogens.

When asked to comment on this the FSANZ (Food Standards Australia and New Zealand) replied that all additives permitted in Australia are considered safe whether or not they are banned overseas!

(For more details and copy of correspondence with the FSANZ see Appendix D).

Here is another example:

Dr. Kaayla Daniel, in her book "The whole Soy Story" indicates levels of soy isoflavones in baby formulas to be many times the safe level.

The oestrogens in soy baby formulas can irreversibly harm the baby's sexual development and reproductive health. Infants fed soy formula take in an estimated five birth control pills worth of oestrogen every day.

I asked a major manufacturer of soy-based baby formulas what amount of soy isoflavones are in their product.

They advised that soy-based infant formulas are approved for use in the Food Standard Code.

(For details of my correspondence with the manufacturer see Appendix E)

Whose advise would you take? Would you carry out your own 'due diligence'?

All decisions made by FSANZ must be approved by a council composed of the Health Minister from each of the Australian states and territories, and the Health Minister from New Zealand, as well as other participating Ministers nominated by each jurisdiction. This has led to political interference in the decision. This is not meant to be a criticism of FSANZ, it is merely an example of a fact which is true of many health regulatory authorities throughout the world. In some countries commercial interests have a major influence on such regulatory decisions.

In the main we are fortunate to have such authorities but when making your decisions it's important to understand that their rulings may be influenced by factors other than our health.

There is an account of how drug companies in the USA influenced the 'cholesterol guidelines' by basing them on information which conflicted with much independent research. As a result of their guidelines there was a marked increase in sales of the drug, statin. On another occasion, a researcher lost his job because he identified homocysteine as a more accurate predictor of heart disease. His findings conflicted with the dogma, of that time, that cholesterol and fats caused heart disease. *(For more details of these two issues see Appendix C).*

An issue that seems to have been muzzled or kept under wraps is the safety of microwaved foods.

Microwaved Foods
Health professionals have records of patients whose health improved once they ceased eating microwaved food. They had been suffering from

headaches, backaches and emotional instability. There is a study to show a significant variation in white blood cells, cholesterol values and haemoglobin after eating microwaved foods. Evidence demonstrates that microwaving breast milk destroys anti-bodies and fosters the growth of potentially pathogenic bacteria.

Experts that issue statements claiming microwaved foods to be safe seem to do so by explaining how the microwaves operate - how they heat food. They conclude that these ovens can therefore do no more damage to foods than that heated in a conventional oven or by cooking.

However, they do not seem interested in testing their theories by finding out what effect eating microwaved food has on a individual's metabolism.

To my mind there is sufficient evidence to cause concern; sufficient evidence for some detailed independent research to be carried out.

Then we have the mixed messages on vitamin supplementation.

Vitamins

There are experts who tell us that vitamins don't work or just contribute to expensive urine!! They have read research on isolated, crystalline or synthetic vitamins and based on that knowledge their advice is often correct. But, do those same people tell us to limit the amount of fruit and vegetables that we eat because we would just end up excreting expensive nutrients!!! Of course they don't.

Let me, however, start this subject on another tack.

The majority of pharmaceutical drugs were initially discovered in plants. There is a story of a major drug manufacturer who, in the middle of last century, sent teams to study the 'recipes' used by West African 'witch doctors' in order to identify plants that might lead them to a useful drug.

The active ingredients identified in these plants are then manufactured in isolation and, after many years research, administered to humans in such concentration as to break through the body's defence system in order to cure the ill from which the patient is suffering. In doing so, however, it invariably causes 'side-effects' which are, hopefully, less severe than the illness.

A similar practice has taken place with vitamins. There are health professionals who recommend isolated vitamins or minerals to counter specific health problems. But Nature does not work that way. Nature works with numerous nutrients having a synergistic effect. Let me give you an example:

An apple contains about 8mg of vitamin C. But the anti-oxidant effect of the whole apple is the equivalent of 1500mg. The vitamin C in isolation is not nearly as effective. It needs to be associated with its cofactors for maximum effect.

When our ancestors were hunter gatherers they roamed the forests and savannahs choosing to eat from some 10,000 different plants. They ate whole plants. The combined nutrients in the whole plants had a synergistic effect. They complimented each other. Nowadays 90% of our nourishment comes from seventeen cultivated species. Many of these we eat after they have been processed, so leaving just a few of the nutrients.

For over 12,000 years - the earliest start of the Agricultural Age - our biochemistry has not changed. We still thrive best on the nutrients with which we evolved.

There are reputed to be somewhere between ten to twenty thousand phytonutrients in plants - maybe even more. They contribute to the wellbeing of the plants that produce them and the animals and humans that eat the plants. Many are anti-oxidants, some act like hormones, and others block the action of cancer producing substances.

These substances are so complex that we may never identify them all, but their interaction is vital to all life processes. It is most unlikely that we will ever know what each one contributes to our health. I am sure that in most cases they do not have a direct influence but they make a synergistic contribution, they improve the performance of nutrients whose specific roles we have already identified.

An example of this is ellagic acid which has been shown to prevent the development of many cancer cells and can destroy the cells themselves. However, synthetic or isolated ellagic acid has potentially serious side-effects one of which is to raise blood pressure; also in its pure form it is not readily biologically available. But, when we eat the whole plant, our intestinal flora hydrolyse their ellagitannins to produce biologically available ellagic acid. This then contributes to prevent the development of cancer cells as well as having anti-bacterial and anti-viral properties. It is only when the whole plant is consumed that the ellagic acid is effective.

The US Agricultural Research Service states: *"In pure form ellagic acid is highly insoluble and biologically unavailable...ellagic acid, as it is biosynthesised in plants, occurs in combination with glucose as elagitannins. These compounds are quite water soluble and biologically available."* The Professor in charge of the trials at the

Cancer Center stated *"it is clear the neutraceutical whole is greater than the sum of its parts".*

The nutrients in plants can build up your immune system. How do vaccinations tie in with this?

Vaccinations

Vaccinations have had a huge impact on the survival and improved lifestyle of millions. But there are obviously concerns in the community about vaccinations. Concerns like do the carriers of the vaccines produce adverse effects and do combinations of vaccines have a synergistically adverse effect. The main thing is that any research can be relied on - it is thorough, unbiased and carried out by independent organisations. At times, particularly when development is rushed, this may be questionable.

Could more effort be expended in promoting foods from healthy soils (biologically fertile) and so improving our health and immune systems?

This leads me to the germ theory and your ecosystem.

The Germ Theory and Bacterial Balance

For generations we have been brought up on Pasteur's "germ theory of disease". Has that narrowed the experts' views of bacteria? Has it prevented medical science from realising that many drugs are opposed to nature's "symbiosis" and have, as a result, been generating new and deadlier varieties of infections?

At the time of Pasteur, the best known biological scientist in France was Professor Béchamp. Briefly, he discovered a "symbiotic" relationship between microbes and larger animals.

He declared that Pasteur was wrong: that the nature of germs was not like higher animals. Microbial life is not firmly set into invariable species. Rather, microbial life is "pleomorphic" - capable of changing form and nature.

However, the orthodox dominating scientific community ignored Béchamp and moved into what became the era of the pathogen hunters and "wonder drugs" that killed the pathogens.

How do these, almost contrasting views, affect your health?

You may be described as an eco-system.

You are host to millions of bacteria which are found in your gut, mouth, all crevices and orifices and on your scalp and skin. With that in mind the two differing views on bacteria become important in making health related decisions.

As a healthy adult you harbour some 100 trillion bacteria, with over 400 different species in your gut alone.

In exchange for raw materials and shelter the microbes, that live in and on you, feed and protect you. So they are integral to your wellbeing. At times, however, this symbiotic arrangement can break down. Then, the microbiome - as your bacteria are collectively known - may cause disease. These diseases tend to be the chronic illnesses that are rife in the rich world. From obesity and diabetes, via heart disease, asthma and multiple sclerosis, to neurological conditions such as autism the microbiome seems to play a crucial role.

As your brain and gut are linked via the nervous system your diet has a powerful influence on your brain health. It can influence depression, anxiety, moods, behaviours, memory and learning.

An 'unbalanced' mix of bacteria can cause problems: The mix of bacteria could cause malnutrition even if the food you consume would otherwise be thought sufficient to sustain you. For instance bacterial enzymes convert carbohydrates called glycans, of which milk has many, into usable sugars. Many such carbohydrates would be indigestible if your digestive system had to work with its own enzymes. So the bacteria use their enzymes for your benefit. You have a symbiotic relationship with bacteria; a relationship which is important in nutrition.

There is a link between the mix of bacteria and the production of an acid that can lead to high blood pressure and so heart disease. A similar mix could be a link to type 2 diabetes. It also seems that some component of the mix confuses the immune system to the detriment of body cells elsewhere. This can be the cause of type 1 diabetes, asthma, eczema and multiple sclerosis.

Danish research indicates that children whose mothers took antibiotics during their pregnancy were more likely to develop asthma than those whose mothers did not take antibiotics? Taking other risk factors into account, researchers estimated that children exposed to antibiotics were 17% more likely to be hospitalised for asthma before age five.

If gut bacteria can make you ill, can changing the mix make you healthy?

There are indications that probiotics, which stimulate the growth of beneficial micro-organisms, can assist. It seems that after a course of antibiotics, which indiscriminately kill beneficial as well as harmful bacteria, eating yogurt or some other form of probiotic for six months can rebalance the mix. However, the yogurt must contain the live culture. But yogurts are limited in the range of bacteria they can transmit.

In really severe cases the gut bacteria have been successfully re-populated by administering an enema of faeces from a healthy person's gut.

Fermented foods are a means to encourage new bacteria growth. They also contain the billions of existing bacteria that have contributed to that fermentation.

One of the best known of these is Sauerkraut or fermented cabbage. The Roman army marched on it; Pliny wrote of ways to make it; Tiberius travelled with a barrel of it on long voyages because he and his fellow Romans knew that it protected them from intestinal infections (due to the lactic acid).

Fermented foods increase your overall nutrition by promoting the growth of friendly intestinal bacteria. These aid digestion and support immune function. They also increase B vitamins , omega-3 fatty acids, digestive enzymes, lactase and lactic acid, and other immune chemicals that fight off harmful bacteria and even cancer cells.

Traditionally fermented foods offer enormous benefit for babies including lowering the risk of adverse vaccine reactions

However, many of today's grocery store varieties of pickles, or fermented foods are acidified and pasteurised for extended shelf life, and as a result, they no longer contain the beneficial bacteria of traditionally fermented foods.

You may enjoy learning simple ways to make your own fermented vegetables. *(Appendix K "Nourishing Traditions")*

What this boils down to is the importance of maintaining a healthy balance of bacteria. When you take antibiotics or drink chlorinated water you are causing species extinction in your gut ecosystem: you are destroying the interdependence found in the mix of the bacteria.

Let's examine salt. You have no doubt heard it is bad for you.

Salt

Some 25 years ago I read of a doctor who used sea salt to lower blood pressure in his patients.

We have been conditioned to believe that salt is bad for us because it causes high blood pressure.

Since the middle of the last century salt consumption in the 'Western World' has almost halved compared to what it was the previous 150 years. This drop was mainly due to refrigeration replacing salt as a main form of food preservation. So why this concern about excess salt?

Salt is essential for good health.

Having evolved from the sea our body's salt to water ratio is critical.

Insufficient salt has been linked to insulin resistance; metabolic syndrome; increased cardiovascular death; cognition loss; unsteadiness, falls, and fractures. The studies identifying health problems with salt would have been carried out with 'table' or 'refined' salt.

In parts of Europe doctors have prescribed sea salt to cure health problems.

What is the difference between Sea Salt and Refined Salt?

Sea Salt has over 80 minerals, whereas refined salt has two. *(For more information Appendix G).*

Just because the label reads 'Sea Salt' it does not mean it hasn't been refined.

Let me reiterate that I do not wish to diminish the work of all experts. My intention is to give a perspective on expert advice which may help you to make your own decisions.

I have briefly covered Nutrition and Disease and explained how Food Manufacturing and Modern Agricultural Practices have affected our health through the foods we consume. I have also discussed the reliability of 'Experts'.

What about sleep? We spend a third of our lives sleeping. How important is that to our health?

SLEEP

Along with nutrition and exercise, good sleep is one of the pillars of health. You cannot achieve optimal health without taking care of your sleep.

Ongoing sleep deficiency can raise the risk for chronic health problems. It has been shown to cause all those diseases known as 'degenerative'. It can affect how well you think, react, work, learn, and get along with others.

If you are sleep deficient you may have trouble making decisions, solving problems, controlling your emotions and behaviour, and coping with change. Sleep deficiency has also been linked to depression, suicide, and risk-taking behaviour.

You need seven to eight hours sleep a night. After several nights of losing sleep - even 1 to 2 hours a night - your ability to function suffers as if you haven't slept at all for a day or two.

In 'The Sleep Revolution' Arianna Huffington writes: "Sleep is a key element of our being and reacts profoundly with each of the other parts. Once I started getting seven or eight hours sleep, it became easier to meditate and exercise, make wiser decisions, and connect more deeply with myself and others".

Where do I see the future?

FUTURE TRENDS

Over the last seventy or more years we have been bombarded with nutritional "health" solutions. Some have caused harm. I see these possible future trends:

- A focus on building up our immune systems - apart from vaccinations.
- An increase in the consumption of fresh foods.
- Major retailers will specify to their suppliers that their produce must come from biologically fertile soils. This might be measured on the Brix Scale. The approach is already under way in South Africa and about to start in the USA. It would provide an improved level of nutrition for the consumer and, for the benefit of the retailer, a longer shelf life for their fruits and vegetables.
- Another trend, which is already noticeable, is 'dig for health', where people have their own vegetable gardens - however small. By making their own compost and adding it to the garden each year they will build up the soil fertility, produce healthy plants and so contribute to their family's health.
- The link between saturated fats, cholesterol and heart disease will continue to be discredited and shown to be a myth. Yet Max Plank's dictum will prevail, namely that "*A new scientific truth does not triumph by convincing its opponents and making them see the light, but rather because its opponents eventually die, and a new generation grows up that is familiar with it*".
- Meanwhile drug companies will continue to promote cholesterol lowering drugs and food manufacturers will continue to promote low fat

foods and include hydrogenated vegetable oils (TFAs) and addictive levels of sugar in their foods.

- Sugar (fructose) will be acknowledged as a major contributor to degenerative diseases.

SO WHAT ARE THE GUIDELINES FOR A HEALTHY LIFE?

There is not one thing, no magic bullet to good health. It is a combination of factors which needs to take into account minor individual differences.

However, in order of priorities I would put nutrition first - eat the 'right' foods from the right source - and then a close second come mental and physical fitness and sleep.

It also helps to have inherited the 'right' genes! However, if we know that we have a family history of a certain disease, we can take action to help prevent those genes expressing themselves. Sometimes what we think may have been inherited through our genes is actually the result of an inherited lifestyle we are duplicating.

Give your children the gift of health. Condition them to a healthy lifestyle by what they see you eat and what you let them eat. Encourage mental and physical exercise. Give them sufficient exposure to sunlight.

Another factor to heed is pollution. We should ensure that the water we drink and the air we breathe are as pristine as possible. Don't let your body be the filter for your tap water and if you are living in a town be aware that there is a much higher than normal incidence of degenerative diseases in people who live within three blocks of a main highway's pollution.

A recent report published in *The Lancet Respiratory Medicine* stated that a fifth of all underweight births can be attributed to pollution. Underweight babies are more likely to suffer from a range of health problems including asthma and heart disease. By moving from a quiet road to a busy one the likelihood of a low birth weight will increase by 18%.

If you wish to know what not to eat, next time you visit a supermarket look at the 'foods' and drinks in the trollies of those who are obviously overweight and on their way to serious health problems.

In writing her book "The Living Soil", which was published in 1943, Lady Eve Balfour included evidence from researchers, explorers, dentists, doctors and anthropologists who described peoples living in isolated areas - people with good health and physique before they had deteriorated after the influx of Western foods. She discovered that it was not the TYPE of food but the SOURCE that made the difference:

- Every edible part in the diet was consumed
- Foods were grown by a system of returning the entire wastes of the community to the soil from which they were produced
- All foods were unprocessed
- The diet started before life began and the parent was as healthy as the child.

These simple steps to good nutrition evolved over thousands of years. But, as our cities expanded, we have become more and more disconnected from Nature. At the same time our food has changed more in the last 40 years than in the previous 40,000 and our bodies cannot adapt that fast.

It reminds me of a story from the Second World War. A young woman from London had arrived to work on a farm in the West of England. As she watched the cows being milked she commented: "Is that where you get your milk? We get ours from a clean dairy".

This 'pyramid' might be a useful set of guidelines in your search for optimal nutrition:

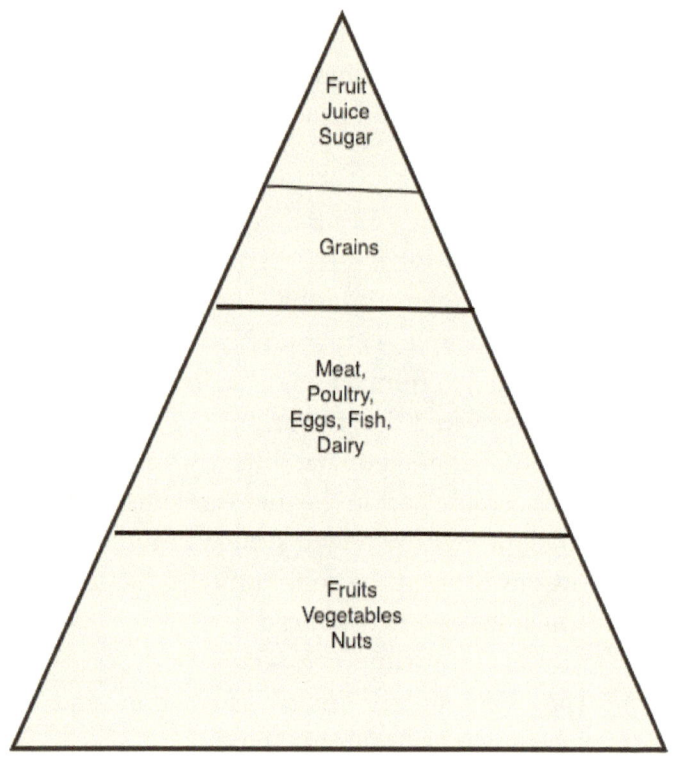

Vegetables

Include a wide variety and have at least one meal a day when you eat them raw, as a salad.

Have as many different colours as possible and include at least 5 different vegetables.

Make your own salad dressing with freshly squeezed lemons, cold pressed olive oil and a mixture of herbs to taste.

If you are steaming vegetables, unless you grow your own, you may find that deep frozen ones have retained a higher level of nutrition.

Include some fermented vegetables with one of your meals.

Nuts
10 to 15 raw nuts a day - (nuts grown on trees).

Fruits
Avoid fruit juice.

You are best to blend the whole fruit so all the fibre remains.

Some apple varieties have been bred to increase the sugar content. British dentists have linked this to a deterioration in children's teeth.

Meat, Poultry, Eggs, Fish, Dairy
Restrict red meat to once a fortnight - pasture fed or wild game.

Cook at low temperatures. Eating meat cooked at high temperatures (300 deg C) or blackening the meat is linked to cancers.

Eat the complete animal - offal as well as muscle meat. This will help keep your homocysteine levels under control.

Best cook with lard, butter, ghee or coconut oil.

Have at least one serving a day of a fermented milk product like yoghurt. Best make your own unless you can establish that what you buy contains live bacteria and no added sugar.

Grains and Sugars
Avoid 'popular' branded breakfast cereals with high sugar content.

Find an organic source of muesli or porridge which has no sugar added.

Eat only sourdough bread.

Restrict to one or two serving of grain-based products a day. (One slice of bread is a serving).

Soak grains overnight to remove anti-nutriuents like phytates.

Organic

Aim to find foods from biologically fertile soils wherever possible. Always ensure that meat comes from livestock grazed on pastures and never from feedlots. (Appendix A)

Avoid farmed fish.

If in doubt stick as close to nature as possible. The less the food has been processed the better.

Salt

It's essential. We need salt. Make sure you use a sea salt with the full range of minerals and no fillers. Avoid refined table salt. *(Appendix G)*

Cooking Tips

- Don't deep fry
- Don't microwave
- If cooking in water make soup out of the liquid or you'll lose most of the nutrients
- Best to sauté, stir fry, or cook with waterless cookware
- Avoid meats barbecued over naked flames or glowing charcoal (these can be carcinogenic)
- Don't cook with vegetable oils. Use butter, coconut oil, ghee or lard.

A Guide To Portion/Serving Sizes

- Your palm in three dimensions, excluding the fingers, is a portion size for meat
- Your fist is a portion size for fruit and vegetables. An apple is about a fist.

- Leafy salads – 2 fists
- One slice bread is one serving

Supplements

By following the above guidelines you will have a healthy plane of nutrition.

However, it is still unlikely that you will have made up for the drop in nutritional value of foods in the last century. In addition, life these days is more stressful and we are exposed to more pollution so in order to attain and maintain optimal health it is wise to take food supplements each day.

In 2002 the Journal of the American Medical Association recommended that we all take vitamin supplements?

Weston Price noted in his travels that even though diets varied considerably the healthy people all ate nutritionally dense foods. The diets *"associated with very high immunity to dental caries and freedom from other degenerative processes"* contained at least four times the level of vitamins and minerals recommended by American nutritionists.

To ensure maximum benefit the supplements must come come from a plant source and these plants should have been grown in biologically fertile soils. Each supplement should contain a plant concentrate. Avoid isolated nutrients - they won't be as biologically available and will not contain the many phytonutrients that provide synergy.

Avoid the mistake of treating food supplements like medicines by taking them when you think you need them. Good food supplements come from healthy plants whence only the fibre and moisture have been removed. The remaining nutrients are available to us as food and like food we need them every day.

Water

Sometimes when you feel hungry it may be thirst. Try drinking a glass of water.

Only drink and cook in water that has been 'purified' by a water filter that complies with international standards (42, 53, 54, 401) and has a device that lets you know when to change the filter. An overdue filter can be more damaging than no filter at all.

Boiling water destroys the bacteria and viruses, not the harmful chemicals. *(Appendix J)*.

Air

If you have someone in the household with respiratory problems or you live in close proximity to a main thoroughfare, instal an air treatment system that will sense the pollution level and automatically turn itself on to filter the air. A good system takes out close on 100% of pollutants.

Sun

Ensure you and your children have the necessary sun exposure. *(See Appendix H)*.

Exercise

Exercise your body and your mind.

Go for a walk five or more days a week and read from a good book or complete a crossword or play a game of scrabble each day. Talk to yourself in a positive way. Learn to use affirmations.

Socialise..........

> Doctor to patient:
> *"What fits your busy schedule better,*
> *exercising one hour a day or being*
> *dead 24 hours a day?"*

Sleep

Make sure you have seven to eight hours sleep a night. It will keep you healthier and make you more productive. Children need up to ten hours a night depending on their age.

Blood and Mineral Analysis

<u>A blood analysis</u> in addition to what your health professional recommends should include:

Vitamin D, Homocysteine, C-reactive protein, Insulin levels, Glucose tolerance.

<u>Mineral analysis</u> Just as a healthy soil requires an optimal balance of minerals so our body requires the same for optimal health. Have an occasional analysis of the mineral levels in your body.

Choosing Your Health Professional

As all diseases are linked to nutrition find a health professional who has an understanding of nutrition over and above what is promoted by government departments. It is advisable to have two opinions. Choose a couple of health professionals in differing disciplines like a GP and a Naturopath.

APPENDICES

APPENDIX A: Milk and Beef

Grass vs Grain

The Weston Price Foundation have published information that shows the difference in quality between milk and butter from dairy cattle that are fed on grain as opposed to fresh grass. Vital nutrients like vitamins A & D and a fat soluble catalyst that promotes optimal mineral assimilation are greatest in milk from cows eating green grass. These nutrients are greatly diminished when cows are fed commercial feed. Vitamins A and D in butterfat are needed for the assimilation of calcium and protein in the water fraction of the milk. Without them protein and calcium are more difficult to utilise and possibly toxic.

Butterfat is rich in short– and medium– chain fatty acids which protect against disease and stimulate the immune system. It contains glyco-spingolipids which prevent intestinal distress and conjugated linoleic acid which has anticancer properties.

Grain fed beef contains excessive amounts of Omega-6 because of the grain and a quarter of the amount of CLA (conjugated linoleic acid) found in pasture fed cattle. CLA has many beneficial properties— it helps prevent atherosclerosis and abnormal blood clotting; limits reactions to allergies; inhibits development of some forms of cancer; stimulates the immune system; has anti-oxidant effects; lowers elevated blood sugar levels; causes cholesterol to become less susceptible to oxidation; helps prevent type 2 diabetes and insulin resistance; assists with weight loss for those classed as obese; lowers triglyceride levels; inhibits the degradation of vitamin E and …..much more.

<u>Pasteurised Milk</u>

In children pasteurised milk has been linked to ear infections, colic, constipation and irritable bowel syndrome, anaemia, nasal congestion, asthma, skin rashes, unexplained vomiting, kidney disease (nephrosis), eczema, anti-social behaviour (young criminals were found to drink almost ten times more milk than the control group).

37% of migraine sufferers have an allergy to it; it can trigger an autoimmune process leading to type 1 diabetes; there is a high correlation between milk consumption Multiple Sclerosis, Lou Gehrig's disease, Crohn's disease and atherosclerosis; it interferes with the body's absorption of manganese and magnesium; it prevents the therapeutic effects of tea polyphenols - *should you therefore add pasteurised milk to your tea?*.

In addition it has been associated with diarrhoea, cramps, bloating and gas, osteoporosis, arthritis, infertility, cancer and dermatitis. No wonder milk is rated as one of the top two allergic foods.

There are, of course, other factors linked to these diseases. The relationship between nutrition and health is complex.

The earlier babies are exposed to pasteurised milk the more likely they are to show signs of intolerances.

Calcium is considered an important constituent of milk. But pasteurisation renders much of the calcium insoluble. Vegetables have greater quantities of calcium.

The Lancet 2001:

Long-term and early -life exposure to stables and (raw) farm milk induces a strong protective effect against the development of asthma, hay fever and atopic sensitisation (rashes).

Journal of Allergy and Clinical Immunology, 2006:
Researchers concluded that children who even infrequently drank raw milk had significantly less current eczema symptoms and a greater reduction in atopy (allergic hypersensitivity)

Clinical and Experimental Allergy, 2007:
Published a study which looked at nearly 15,000 children between the ages of five and thirteen. Researchers found that consumption of raw milk was the strongest factor in reducing the risk of asthma and allergy, a stronger factor than living on a farm or having a pet.

A1 & A2 Milk

A1 milk is linked to higher rates of heart attacks, autism, multiple sclerosis, schizophrenia and deaths from mental disorders. There are also many instances of people who get allergies from A1 milk and not A2. So it is not just a lack of the lactose enzyme that causes milk allergies. In 'The Devil in the Milk' Professor Keith Woodford states: 'The beta-casein proteins found in cattle comprise 209 amino acids in a fixed sequence and making up a convoluted string. The difference between the A1 and A2 variants is just one of these 209 amino acids'.

APPENDIX B: Essential Fatty Acids (EFA's)

Here is a potted summary of the benefits of Omega-3:
- Ensures cell membranes are flexible and contain large numbers of insulin receptors that are more receptive and responsive to circulating

insulin. This results in decreased fat storage in the 'fat cells'

- Turn on the fat burning genes and turn off the fat storage genes.
- Diminish C-reactive proteins: high levels are a risk factor associated with inflammatory diseases such as atherosclerosis, angina, coronary heart disease, heart attack, stroke, congestive heart failure and diabetes.
- Ability to reduce blood pressure.
- Pain management from reduced inflammation. Good for those suffering from arthritis.
- EPA regulates blood supply to the brain which helps concentration. DHA is important in brain membranes: it assists memory and increases serotonin levels (the happy neurotransmitter). This decreases the incidence of depression and anxiety.
- Improve cardiovascular risk profile by lowering VLDL, triglycerides, homocysteine, fibrinogen and increasing HDL - 'good cholesterol' - levels. Combined with various plant nutrients these levels improve even more.
- Assists in reducing the effects of stress by reducing the hormones produced as a result of stress.

<u>Omega-3's effects on children</u>

Long-term studies show that children of women who had consumed the smallest amounts of omega-3 during their pregnancies had verbal IQ's six points lower than average.

If this were widespread it would have a serious effect on a country's brain power.

The second finding was that at three years old, those children with the best measure of fine-motor performance were the ones whose mothers had had the highest intake of omega-3s.

The researchers also found that a low intake of omega-3s during pregnancy led to higher levels of pathological social interactions such as the inability to make friends.

<u>Omega-3's effects on the behaviour of adults</u>

One study shows that omega-3 supplements given to violent alcoholics reduced their anger levels by a third within three months. This study concentrated on omega-3 intake directly. But there is a second way that its level may be reduced—by competition with omega-6. The ratio of omega-3 to omega-6 in the cell membranes – particularly nerve cells— is at the root of the problem, since that can affect the ability of messenger molecules to pass through the membrane.

<u>In summary</u>

Lack of Omega 3 is directly linked to Heart Attacks, Coronary Artery Disease, Atherosclerosis, Stroke, Crohn's Disease, Cancer (Breast, Colon, Prostrate), Obesity, Insulin Resistance, Diabetes, Asthma, Lupus, Rheumatoid Arthritis, Depression, Schizophrenia, Attention Deficit, Hypertension, Hyperactivity, Post Partum Depression, Alzheimer's Disease.

There are, of course, other factors which also affect most of these.

APPENDIX C: "Cholesterol Guidelines"

The following is quoted from 'Modern Nutritional Diseases' (February 2003) by Alice Ottoboni PhD and Fred

Ottoboni MPH, PhD. Both were involved in public health for most of their working lives.

As presented to the public, these new guidelines appear to be written and promoted by a branch of the US Government.....but the facts suggest something different....they were written by a non-government organisation....a sub-group called the Expert Panel on Detection, Evaluation, and Treatment of High Blood Cholesterol in Adults. This Expert Panel was composed primarily of experts from the drug industry......this approach suggests a strategy in which special interests use the stature and credibility of a government agency to promote faulty science that supports the sale of vegetable oils, low fat, low-cholesterol foods and certain prescription drugs.

A research scientist and reviewer of literature on diet, cholesterol and cardiovascular disease wrote:

'Not only does the panel exaggerate the risk of coronary disease and the relevance of high cholesterol, it also ignores a wealth of contradictory evidence. The panel statements reveal that its members have little clinical experience and lack basic knowledge of medical literature or, worse, they ignore or misquote all studies that contradict their view.'

Skyrocketing statin drug sales evidence that the nation's medical professionals are responding to the guidelines.

Scientific literature indicates that an elevated blood level of homocysteine is a more accurate predictor of heart disease than is a high cholesterol level..........this linkage was discovered by Kilmer McCully. Because his findings conflicted with the dogma of that time, namely that cholesterol and fats caused heart disease, he lost his research position at a university hospital and was shunned for some years by the academic community.

McCully's original findings have since been confirmed by many research papers.

APPENDIX D: "Food Colourings and Preservatives"
It is estimated that an average Australian consumes five kilograms of food additives each year.

The good news is that most of these are considered to be quite safe....however...

- Some 50 of these 'approved' chemical additive are known to cause behavioural changes in children & adolescents.

- Many of these additives are also known to cause severe allergic reactions including rashes, headaches, migraines & asthma to name a few.

- Research is showing substantial links between the use of certain food additives and the increase in physical and behavioural health problems in our society.

- Additives, are only tested in isolation. They are not tested in any combinations with other additives. The effect of combining four common additives were observed (aspartame, brilliant blue, msg & quinoline yellow). This study indicated that the additives stopped the nerve cells from growing and interfered with proper signalling systems!!

The body responsible for approving these additives is the Food Standards Australia and New Zealand (FSANZ).

The Quality Control Manager of a world-leading fast food chain posed the following questions to the FSANZ:

"Why in Australia do we have additives that are prohibited in other countries as being suspected or known carcinogens?"

Their answer:

"Different countries have different approval systems. Some countries ban products if they cause DNA changes at any level in any animal.....just because something causes cancer in rats doesn't mean it will cause cancer in humans"

QC manager:

"But what about something like Amaranth (123) – a banned carcinogen in the US that is still permitted in Australia?"

Their answer:

"The US has a different system – all additives permitted in Australia are considered safe whether or not they are banned overseas. I cannot comment on other countries systems."

APPENDIX E: "Soy in baby formula"

Dr. Kaayla Daniel, in her book "The whole Soy Story" indicates levels of soy isoflavones in baby formulas to be many times the safe level.

The oestrogens in soy baby formulas can irreversibly harm the baby's sexual development and reproductive health. Infants fed soy formula take in an estimated five birth control pills' worth of oestrogens every day.

I had asked a major manufacturer of soy-based baby formulas what amount of soy isoflavones are in their product. As a result of their reply I emailed them:

Thank you for the message from your Scientific team. It concerns me.

You state that you ensure that your baby formula quality assurance meets your stringent requirements yet you claim to have no idea what the level of soy isoflavones are in your products - it is apparently not part of your analytical testing.

Do your scientists know that amounts of 0.6mg to 0.75mg isoflavones per kg of body weight causes thyroid suppression and hormonal changes (endocrine disruption) in adults? Please ask them to advise me what they consider to be safe levels for babies and if they do not test for isoflavones how do they know they are within the safe levels?

I received the following reply:

Further to your email regarding soy isoflavones, our Scientific and Regulatory team have provided the following response.

Isoflavones are present in soybeans and soybean products. There has been a long history of safe use of soy in infant formula. The Food Standards Australia New Zealand (FSANZ) is the government agency responsible for developing and administering the Australia New Zealand Food Standards Code, which lists requirements for foods such as additives, food safety, labelling and GM foods. Soy-based infant formulas are approved for use in the Food Standards Code.

(An example of how to answer a question without answering it).

APPENDIX F: "GM Foods"

According to documents released from a lawsuit, scientists at the FDA warned that GM foods might create allergies, poisons, new diseases, and nutritional problems. The White House ordered the agency to promote biotechnology, and Michael Taylor, Monsanto's former attorney, headed up the FDA's GMO policy.

That policy declares that no safety studies on GMOs are required. Monsanto and other producers determine if their foods are safe.

Taylor later became Monsanto's vice president, and was reinstalled at the FDA in 2009 by the Obama administration as the US Food Safety Czar.

Soon after GM soy was introduced to the UK, soy allergies skyrocketed by 50 percent. Ohio allergist Dr. John Boyles says: "I used to test for soy allergies all the time, but now that soy is genetically engineered, it is so dangerous that I tell people never to eat it."

In 2009, the American Academy of Environmental Medicine called for a moratorium on GM foods, and said that long-term independent studies must be conducted, stating:

"Several animal studies indicate serious health risks associated with GM food, including infertility, immune problems, accelerated ageing, insulin regulation, and changes in major organs and the gastrointestinal system. ...There is more than a casual association between GM foods and adverse health effects. There is causation..."

APPENDIX G: "Salt"

Sea salt contain 92 essential minerals and most refined sea salts contain only 2 elements (Na and Cl). Biologically, 24 of the elements in real sea salt have already been proven necessary and essential to maintain and recover health. See Scientific American, July 1972: "The Chemical Elements of Life," by Earl Friden.

Natural sea salt allows liquids to freely cross body membranes, the kidney's glomerulus and blood vessels walls. Whenever the sodium chloride concentration rises in the blood, the water in the neighbouring tissues is attracted to that salt-rich blood, and the cells then re-absorb the enriched intra-cellular fluid. If they are functioning properly, the kidneys remove the saline fluids easily.

Refined salt does not allow this free-crossing of liquids and minerals, and as a result causes accumulated fluids to stagnate, producing oedema and chronic kidney problems. To prevent any moisture from being re-absorbed, the salt refiners add aluminosilicate of sodium or yellow prussiate of soda as desiccants plus different bleaches to the final salt formula. After these processes, the table salt will no longer combine with human body fluids and causes problems such as oedema (water retention) amongst other things.

Real sea salt has the ability to naturally alter or change one element or nuclide into another item as needed.

Salt is the single element required for the proper breakdown of plant carbohydrates into useable and assimilable human food. Only when salt is added to fruits and vegetables can saliva and gastric secretions readily break down the fibrous store of carbohydrates. In the UK, when salt was removed from many of the school lunches, students avoided their salads and vegetables until they got home where they were allowed to sprinkle them with salt which made them more palatable

Sea salt bears a likeness to human blood and body fluids. During World War II when blood supplies ran out, Navy doctors are reputed to have used sea salt water for blood transfusions.

The following information is mostly from Dr. Jacques de Langre, a California biochemist who studied the health benefits of salt for over 35 years. His Ph.D. is in biochemistry from the University of Brussels. He wrote two books on this topic, "Sea Salt's Hidden Powers" and "Sea Salt, the Vital Spark for Life":

- Refined salt (pure sodium chloride) is toxic to the body - and can cause high blood pressure. Celtic sea salt is extremely healthy, and has the exact opposite effect of refined salt.
- If your tears weren't salty, if your sweat wasn't salty...you wouldn't be functioning very well. You can't function without salt. Healthy organ function is depending on good quality nutrition. Good quality Sodium is the predominant cation in circulating blood plasma and tissue fluids. People forget everyone was born in a saline solution, our Mother's amniotic fluid. This is probably the best biological proof we have that the cellular structure is enhanced by salt.
- A low-salt diet can actually cause high blood pressure in some people. A salt-free diet can damage the valves of the heart. The heart can no longer contract normally. Remember, the heart is fed by a saline solution from the blood and lymph.
- On a salt-free diet, the valves of the heart can tire. They will begin to lacerate, and break up in shreds. Without salt, the cells starve. On a salt-free diet, you will not recover quickly after an illness.
- If salt was so bad, why do they feed intravenous saline solutions to hospital patients? They do that because the body runs on salt. Without salt, we run out of electrolytes. Without electrolytes, our human batteries die out.
- Most sea salt can be just as bad for your health as regular salt, because it is so highly refined. You can tell sea salt is refined if it does not have any sign of moisture at all. Refined salt is very

dry salt. This tells you the magnesium has been taken out, because magnesium is a water-hugging molecule.

- Vegetables cannot be fully digested without being salted. When you use the Celtic salt, I would say you can get up to seven times the nutrition out of vegetables. For example, take leeks or dandelion roots. They are supposed to be a good diuretic. If you don't use any Celtic salt, dandelion root really acts very little on the urinary tract. But put a little Celtic salt on it and the potency is vastly increased.

- When someone starts using Celtic Sea Salt the response is a renewal of energy. Fatigue diminishes. You also have more mental alertness. As for adverse reactions, some people get rashes. The salt acts as a scavenger and purges the body of many toxins. These toxins come out into the circulatory and lymph system and particularly the kidney area. This is where the rash comes from; it is a cleansing of the kidney. This is a normal reaction for people who have many toxins. If you are not toxic, it will not happen. A similar reaction is that sores will break out under the armpits. If you do take the Celtic salt and you do get a rash, you can say, "Hallelujah", something good is happening to me. When that happens, all you have to do is take baths with the Celtic salt and rub the rash very gently with the saline solution. This will get the skin to function as an elimination organ. After the mild rash has gone, warts and black skin moles have been known to shrink, shed and drop off.

de Langre makes the following summary:

- A low-salt diet for the treatment of high blood pressure is based on dogma, not evidence
- A salt restrictive diet can actually RAISE your blood pressure
- A lack of salt can cause accelerated ageing, cellular degeneration and biochemical starvation
- A lack of salt can cripple your health and cause liver failure, kidney problems and massive adrenal exhaustion
- On a salt-free diet, the valves of your heart muscle can tire, lacerate and cause a fatal heart attack

APPENDIX H: "Sun Exposure"

Colin Campbell, Professor Emeritus, Cornell University recommends:

"If you know how much sunshine causes a redness of your skin, then one third of this amount, provided two to three times per week, is more than adequate to meet our Vitamin D needs and to store some in our liver and body fat. If your skin becomes slightly red after about thirty minutes in the sun, then ten minutes, three times per week will be enough exposure to get plenty of Vitamin D".

Also check the Cancer Council website:

http://www.cancer.org.au/preventing-cancer/sun-protection/vitamin-d/

'dminder.info' is a very helpful app

APPENDIX J: "Water"

Summary of a report in a South Australian newspaper:

Freedom of Information data from SA Water shows the state's tap water breached the Australian Drinking Water Guidelines or World Health Organisation guidelines 9298 times between January 2000 and July 2012.

While Government authorities say South Australians have nothing to fear, experts say it is unclear whether prolonged exposure would increase the risk of cancer.

The Cancer Council also said some animal studies had shown a link between the chemicals and some cancers.

Researcher Anthony Amis said:

'the most worrying breaches related to the potentially cancer causing by-products from the chlorine disinfection process, which was used to rid the water of harmful micro-organisms......These by-products, called trihalomethanes (THMs), form when the chlorine reacts with organic matter in the water.

There are four THMs which, when tested as a group, should not exceed 250 parts per billion.

If these compounds were calculated individually, there were almost 3000 individual disinfection by-product breaches. People with compromised immune systems have to be really careful about drinking chlorinated water.

The main compounds the WHO are concerned about are the higher risk of bladder cancer and there could be slight rises in reproductive disorders as well'.

The reason for including the above is to emphasise the THMs which are produced as a result of chlorine reacting with organic matter. This happens <u>after the water leaves the processing plant.</u>

APPENDIX K: The China Study by T. Colin Campbell

I found The China Study an exciting read. It was well written. But after thinking about the author's comments that linked animal proteins to cancer, and his advise to adopt a vegan diet, it did not make sense when I considered the historical evidence. I wrote him a letter asking for his comments to thirteen questions but in spite of follow up emails I never received a reply.

I mention this as an example of being initially convinced by a well written book from a very credible author; but which on subsequent reflection seems to have reached some questionable conclusions. Subsequently, I learnt others have pointed out flaws in his information.

Here are the questions I asked him to which I never received a reply:

1. In the cold climates of the north peoples have evolved as mainly meat eaters. To your knowledge is there a higher incidence of degenerative diseases in these populations than elsewhere?

    There are also tribes like the Masai in East Africa who drink a mixture of cows' blood and milk. Yet they appear to be very healthy.

    The Australian aborigine, before the advent of the western diet, consumed 30% to 60% of their diet as meat – kangaroo, goanna (and other lizards), wombat, emu and, on the coast and along some rivers, fish. The variation depended on which area of Australia.

    In "The Stuff Man's Made Of " the author summarises reports of researchers and explorers, dentists, doctors and anthropologists who studied people living in isolated areas, who had good health and physique, before they had access to 'Western Foods'. He wrote that their reports bring out three significant points:

    a. These communities lived arduously and frugally under exacting and at times harsh conditions; yet they suffered from none of the physical and nervous disorders now so rife amongst "civilised" communities. The little they had of food resources seems to have resulted in a considerably higher plane of nutrition and health than does the much that we have.

b. They represented the widest conceivable variety of race, climatic and topographical environment, and diet, the latter ranging from lacto-vegetarian to almost wholly carnivorous.

c. The one thing they do seem to have had in common was the unsophisticated nature of their foods and the fact that they consumed these whole, ie. Without discarding any edible portions.

In 'The Living Soil' Lady Eve Balfour wrote:
"the Hunza tribe on the extreme northern frontier of India, superb and exceptionally thrifty agriculturists, living on cereals, pulse, fruit, vegetables, milk and a little meat; the islanders of the Faroes, Iceland, and Greenland, living mainly on wild animals, birds and fish; the Polar Eskimos, living on seals and sea-birds and their eggs; the people of Tristan da Cunha living on fish and potatoes, with some milk and seabirds' eggs; the North American Indians, hunters of the prairies and forests; and the Chinese of certain rural areas, some of the thriftiest and most intensive agriculturists in the world."
…"The only discernable common factor, other than good air, seems to be that the diets of all these groups are 'whole' diets in the full sense of the word. That is to say:

a. Every edible part in the diet was consumed – the whole grain or animal

b. Foods were grown by a system of returning the entire wastes of the community to the soil from which they were produced (this could be land, sea or lake).

 c. All foods were unprocessed

 d. The diet started before life began and the parent was as healthy as the child.

So it seems from these observations that it was not the TYPE of food but the SOURCE that made the difference.

In "Health Secrets of the Stone Age" Philip Goscienski quotes from scores of studies of ancient and modern hunter gatherer societies which show that Stone Age Man consumed 33% protein v's 12% for contemporary Americans - a bit lower than your figure. So Stone Age Man consumed 2 to 3 times the proportion of protein to modern man.

 a. Could it be that our modern farming methods have changed the constituents of the foods more than merely the content of the macro and micro-nutrients?

 b. Did you notice any difference in your China Study between the health of those who relied mainly on foods/animal proteins produced by 'traditional methods' (China has had a long tradition of composting) compared to those who ate foods produced mainly through 'modern/high yield/scientific' methods?

 c. Just as your research indicates a difference between animal and plant protein, could there be a difference between animal proteins depending on that animal's nutrition?

 d. Have you noted a difference between people who drink pasteurised milk v's fresh whole milk?

e. These days milk is one of the two major food allergies. It seems to have commenced when high yielding dairy cattle (like Friesians) were fed 'concentrates' to increase yields. (I think one has to expect problems when one feeds ruminants anything but fodder on pastures). Could the casein that you used for your rats have come from these and might that have made a difference?

f. Is there a difference in the health of peoples in China eating meat from wild or range fed animals as opposed to lot (grain) fed animals?

g. Your population sample in the China Study came from the same gene pool (likewise, presumably the rats in your laboratory studies). Is it possible that peoples who survive mainly on meat could have evolved to make use of animal proteins without the harmful effects that you have identified?

2. It seems that homo sapiens may well have overtaken the other species of homo through extra consumption of omega 3. Most of this extra consumption would have come from fish. Since the start of the agricultural age, some 11,000 years ago man's brain has shrunk about 10% - quite likely as a result of consuming ever decreasing amounts of omega 3.

Was there any difference in the China Study (or any other that you are aware of) between the health of those who obtained their animal protein from fish v's other sources?

3. I am interested in your concern about GM foods. Apart from the possible ecological problems, as far as I know there is no requirement for the instigators

of GM crops to prove safety to humans....yet for drugs they are required to do so.

The two main food allergies are milk and wheat. I understand a reason for wheat being an allergy is that modern wheats contain 22 genes, whereas the original varieties contained 9.

Modern man has not evolved enough to cope with the extra genes. If we have such a reaction to plants bred fairly naturally it concerns me what can happen with plants that are genetically engineered the 'modern' way.

4. Have you noted any difference in the health of two groups of peoples consuming similar amounts of animal proteins but different amounts of 'plants'? In other words can the extra plants counteract the damage done by animal protein?

5. Since it appears that carcinogens have to be 'activated' by animal proteins, is there any evidence from your study that smokers who consume a mainly plant based diet have considerably less lung cancer than those who consume a mainly meat diet?

6. You state that eating foods containing any cholesterol above 0 mg is unhealthy.
    Alice Ottoboni PhD and Fred Ottoboni MPH, PhD, in the summary of their book "The Modern Nutritional Diseases" state that 'Dietary cholesterol is not absorbed well from the intestinal tract, and whatever amount is absorbed merely reduces the amount of cholesterol the body needs for itself. Thus cholesterol present in foods does not have a significant effect on blood cholesterol levels. On the other hand certain dietary regimes that force the

body to make more cholesterol than it requires do result in excess cholesterol in the blood. A diet excessively high in carbohydrate calories, particularly sugars and refined starches, is such a regime.

'..Except in rare cases of familial hypercholesterolemia, excess cholesterol in the blood is the result of excess dietary sugar and starch'.

Is this relevant to your findings?

I understand that hypercholesterolemia is a genetic defect. Do you know the incidence of this in the Chinese population?

7. I am interested in your comments about vitamin supplementation. There is much research on micro nutrients that appears to be contradictory. I always have to remind myself that I must get away from the trees and see what makes sense as part of the forest - what happens in Mother Nature. If it does not match my understanding of that, then, I question the evidence.

I have for some time been intrigued by the way naturopaths seem to be going the way of the 'conventional' medical profession in that they recommend individual vitamins for specific ailments. They are in fact treating them like the 'conventionals' prescribe drugs.

What is your opinion of the AMAJ (2002) advice that all adults should take a multi vitamin supplement?

You comment on the beta carotene studies with smokers. I assume you are referring to the Oxford and Helsinki studies. A cardiologist in Sydney, who has been very successful in reversing his patients' problems (to the scorn of his colleagues), has commented, that these studies were carried out with synthetic beta-carotene. This breaks down easily. When it does break down it turns into a virulent free radical. As the smokers were not advised to change their lifestyle – they continued smoking – this would have hastened the breakdown of the synthetic beta-carotene and helped to cause the increase in lung cancer.

This is another example of using isolated vitamins like a drug.

Have you heard of Carl Rehnborg?

In China during the 1920's he noticed a link between health and nutrition. Health varied with the consumption of various plant foods and the degree to which they were processed (eg polished rice compared to unhusked). He had the idea that if you had a healthy soil, the plants growing in it would be healthy and this would be passed on to the peoples eating those plants. To get those healthy plants to as many people as possible, he spent some years working out how to take the fibre and moisture out of these plants and encapsulate the remaining nutrients. He launched his product in 1934 and it has been marketed under the Nutrilite brand.

I was fascinated when I first visited their farm in California thirty years ago......here was a man who had had a similar idea to Friend Sykes and the same time! Whereas Friend Sykes marketed his crops, Carl Rhenborg concentrated his crops before marketing them. His products have always had the complete plant concentrate in them.

Nutrilite has independent clinical studies carried out on its formulations. Last year they published one which showed a rapid reduction in DNA fragmentation in the subjects who ate the Nutrilite product.

Through their farming techniques they have learnt how to increase the plants' phytonutrients content up to tenfold. You might be interested in their farming methods – their website gives a preliminary account.

8. I understand there is some doubt about the health benefits of soy unless it is fermented. Is there any support for this in your China project?

9. Did you note any difference in the nutritional value of the same crops in different areas or under different farming methods in China? If so was there any difference in the health of the population?

10. Did you notice any difference in the health of the Chinese populations depending on their cooking methods or between those that ate more raw foods than cooked?

11. A major prolonged trauma early in life affects one's hormonal system so that it can lead to chronic diseases in later life. The current population of China have gone through the 'Great Leap Forward', 'The Great Famine', and the 'Cultural Revolution'. Different regions were affected to a different extent. Was any of this noticeable in the China Study?

12. Your chart 4:9 'Plant fat intake and breast cancer' shows that Spain and Greece have about the same or greater intake of vegetable oils than USA, Switzerland and the Netherlands yet their death rates are way below. Could this have something to do with the fact that Greece and Spain would get

most of their vegetable oils from olive oil and the others would get theirs from grains like canola, sunflower and corn? I have always wondered whether tree crops should be classed as vegetables! In other words olive oil, coconut oil, and oils from other nuts are probably different from vegetable oils that come from annual crops.

There seems to be evidence that those grown on trees do not hydrogenate – although I have heard conflicting evidence of this as far as olive oil is concerned. However, if I am correct in the above interpretation of your chart it seems to confirm that there is a difference.

13. You mention that a vegan diet can cure type 2 diabetes. If someone already has insulin resistance, how is a diet high in complex carbohydrates going to reduce this resistance when grains (very dense carbs), for example, need lots of insulin to break them down? Are you referring to any vegan diet or one that avoids plants with dense carbs?

    (Here is a comment from a friend which is relevant to this: "I have seen cases where insulin resistance has been controlled to the point where people no longer need any medication.

    The general rule seems to be lots of low density carbs such as non starchy fruit and vegetables with a small portion of protein at main meals. This seems to be easier to achieve with animal proteins as most plant based protein sources (apart from tofu) are relatively carbohydrate dense, whereas with animal proteins there are no carbs and hence no insulin response. This pattern decreases the insulin response and at the same time the protein seems to reduce the hunger pangs").

APPENDIX L: Reading Matter

Here is some of the material that has helped stimulate my thinking on nutrition and health. I don't necessarily agree with everything in all the books. I have many others in my library on these subjects but I have not considered them worth listing.

Seeds of Deception	Jeffrey M. Smith
The Untold Story of Milk	Ron Schmid ND
Modern Nutritional Diseases	Alice Ottoboni PhD and Fred Ottoboni MPH, PhD
The Cell Factor	Dr Ross Walker
The Omega Plan	Artemis P. Simopoulos MD
Health Secrets of the Stone Age	Dr Philip Goscienski
The Stuff Man's Made Of	Jorian Jenks
Modern Humus Farming	Friend Sykes
The China Study	Colin Campbell (see appendix K)
Essays, Speeches, Writings.	C.F. Rehnborg
Devil in the Milk	Keith Woodford
Dr Atkins New Diet Revolution	Robert C.Atkins MD
Sweet Poison	David Gillespie
The Whole Soy Story	Kaayla Daniel PhD, CCN
The Biogenic Diet	Leslie Kenton
Immune System	Dr Bruce Miller DDS CNS
The Water Your Drink	John Archer
Fit for Life	Harvey & Marilyn Diamond
Life - An unauthorised biography	Richard Fortey
The Earth - A Intimate History	Richard Fortey
The Secret Life of Trees	Colin Tudge
The Ascent of Man	Jacob Bronowski
Nourishing Traditions	Sally Fallon & Mary Enig Ph.D
Death by Food Pyramid	Denise Minger
The Living Soil	E.B. Balfour
The Sleep Revolution	Arianna Huffington

EPILOGUE

Many of the emphases in this book are mine. Occasionally quotes or statements contradict each other - I think it clear which I support. If in doubt try to go back to basics - ask yourself 'what might Nature's response be?' I hope the information stimulates you to form your own views and that these will contribute to your health.

The way you treat your health now will have a major effect on your health in ten to fifteen years time.

Once you've decided on your own health plan, stick to it. Don't let anything deter you from it. Remember - it's only your health that is at stake!

Frank Tennant
December 2014
Revised January 2016
Revised June 2017